Book 1
Essential Oils & Aromatherapy for Beginners
BY LINDSEY P

&

Book 2
The Beginners Guide to Medicinal Plants

BY LINDSEY P

Book 1
Essential Oils & Aromatherapy for Beginners

BY LINDSEY P

Secrets to Beauty, Health and Weight Loss Using Proven
Essential Oil and Aromatherapy Recipes

2nd Edition

Essential Oils Box Set #33: Essential Oils & Aromatherapy for Beginners & The Beginners Guide to Medicinal Plants

Table Of Contents

Introduction

I want to thank you and congratulate you for purchasing the book, *"Essential Oils & Aromatherapy for Beginners: Secrets to Beauty, Health and Weight Loss Using Proven Essential Oil and Aromatherapy Recipes ".*

This book contains proven steps and strategies on how to use essential oils, either pure or in combination, to solve common problems in beauty and health. Using essential oils as opposed to commercial formulations for your various problems can help you maintain an all-natural lifestyle. This is good for the environment, for yourself and, in certain circumstances, for your wallet too.

Thanks again for purchasing this book, I hope you enjoy it!

Chapter 1 -- Using Essential Oils

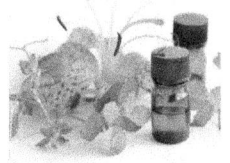

Essential oils have been used for centuries in many cultures to cure common health ailments, solve various household problems, soothe the soul, make someone fall in love with you, drive evil spirits away and many others. While some of these uses may have been proven false by science, many are retained particularly for beauty and over-all health.

Technically speaking, an essential oil is the oily liquid that is distilled from the whole plant or certain parts of it. The color, oiliness and viscosity of an essential oil vary depending on the plant. Some essential oils feel like water and are as clear as water while some will feel oily and will have a yellowish or brownish color.

Essential oils are given that name because they are, in a sense, the essence of the plant. Think of them as the concentrated goodness of the plant. This is why they ought to be used sparingly and also why they can, especially for topical uses, be good for your wallet. Depending on the brand and on the essential oil, a 30 ml. bottle will usually cost around US $20, but since you only use 1 to 2 drops at a time, that small bottle will go a long way.

Essential oils will have their own scent and are commonly used in making fragrance, but they should be differentiated from fragrance oils which are artificially scented oils. The latter are commonly used in oil burners, for potpourri and sometimes for cheap scented soaps and candles. To the uninitiated, fragrance oils and products made with them can seem like a better buy because they are cheaper, but there will be a difference in the scent of true essential oil and artificial fragrance oil. The longer you have used true essential oils, the more you can distinguish between them and artificial scents.

Some proponents of aromatherapy will insist that only true essential oils will give actual benefits. This is debatable since there have been no serious studies made on this yet. If you are using fragrance oils for your oil burner or for making candles because they are cheaper, and you think the scent is giving you some benefits, then by all means continue to use this fragrance oil. However, I will encourage you to splurge on true essential oil to learn the difference. Soon, you might find that true essential oil gives you better benefits and you will find that the difference in cost is worth it.

Fragrance oils can be used safely for oil burners and scenting potpourri, BUT they should never be used topically on the skin. Some cheap kinds of soaps which are scented with fragrance oils may not irritate the skin since only a small amount is used, but if you use pure fragrance oils directly on the skin, even the most insensitive skins can experience irritation. Also, since fragrance oils are only artificially scented oils, you will not get any skin care benefits from them as you would from true essential oils.

If cost is really a problem with essential oils, you should know that they are concentrated and are usually used diluted with vegetable oil. This is commonly called 'carrier oil' because they 'carry' the essential oil. The best carrier oils are those which do not have a natural scent like jojoba or grape seed oil. These oils also feel light on the skin since they have a similar composition to sebum or our skin's natural oil. For drier skins, olive, rose hip, coconut or avocado oil may be better options but they can have a natural scent of their own and can affect the overall scent of your essential oil. We will further discuss carrier oils per se in chapter 4.

You need to experiment on the right ratio of essential oil and carrier oil for your specific skin type. Always start with a 1:1 ratio then add more carrier oil if you experience irritation or add more essential oil if you are not seeing the results you want.

Always keep your essential oils in a cool dark place regardless whether they are diluted or pure. Take note that most essential oils are stored in dark bottles. As much as possible, when making your own combinations, use dark bottles as well. Also, it is better to buy small amounts of essential oil and wait until this is used up before buying a new one. This way you can be assured that the essential oil you use is always fresh.

The potency of essential oils must always be stressed since you might hurt yourself if you are not careful. Certain essential oils can also be extremely irritating to the eyes and mouth when they are used near these areas. Those with sensitive skins must be particularly careful because they can still experience irritation even when essential oils are used diluted.

Also, it is possible to be allergic to essential oils. If you have a lot of allergies, it is better to do a skin test first before using the essential oil for your topical skin care. If you will not use the essential oil for topical purposes, then you need not do a skin test.

To do a skin test, apply a small drop of the pure essential oil on a hidden part of the body like the inside of your elbow. Wait for 24 hours to see if any redness or irritation will happen. If you do not experience irritation, you can safely use the essential oil for skin and health care. You should do this for every essential oil you need to use.

There are some who say that even if you experience irritation with the pure oil, you can still use it diluted. If you wish to test this on yourself, do the same skin test described above but dilute the small drop of pure essential oil with the same amount of your choice of carrier oil. However, do not risk doing this if you have extremely sensitive skin.

The succeeding chapters will teach you which essential oils are the best for many problems. It might seem as if you need to buy several bottles of various kinds, but if you read carefully, you will notice that one essential oil can have various uses. For example, lavender essential oil can be used for acne, for calming the mind, for wrinkles and for minor skin burns. Thus, if you are already using this for your acne, you can use the same bottle for other purposes as well.

This can be another reason why it is better to buy true essential oil instead of fragrance oils even if you initially had no intention of using the fragrance oil topically. If you bought a cheap bottle of lavender fragrance oil, you can only use this for scenting your room, and it will be an inferior scent at that. If you buy true lavender essential oil, the whole family can use that single bottle *and* you get a better scent.

Chapter 2 – Skin Care

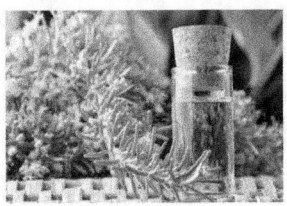

There are various skin care problems which essential oils can cure. The most common are acne, wrinkles or aging skin, fungal infections, psoriasis and eczema, and minor skin burns and wounds. We will discuss each problem in turn.

For acne, the most effective essential oils are tea tree oil, lavender and neem oil. These essential oils effectively kill acne bacteria. Depending on the severity of your acne and the sensitivity of your skin, use the pure essential oil or appropriately diluted. The lighter vegetable oils like jojoba and grape seed are the better choice for oily skins, but if you have normal or dry skin and just happen to suffer from acne, coconut oil can be a good choice since it can add anti-bacterial properties to your essential oil solution.

What you choose will depend on how fast you wish your acne to be gone and your scent preference. Tea tree oil is generally considered the fastest acting essential oil for acne followed by lavender oil and neem oil. However, take note that even tea tree oil will act slower compared to commercial acne treatments containing benzoyl peroxide and salicylic acid. If so, what can be a reason for you to choose essential oils? As mentioned in the introduction, you can opt to choose essential oils because you prefer a natural lifestyle. Also, in the long run, essential oils can be cheaper because you use only a very small amount.

Regarding scent, tea tree oil is spicy and woody, lavender is soothing and feminine while neem oil is the worst smelling. The scent of neem oil has been compared to a skunk and to stale urine, but it has an added benefit of smoothing out fine lines and wrinkles. Thus, if you have mature skin and suffer from acne, neem oil can be the better option. The scent can be minimized by your carrier oil and by a small amount of either lavender or tea tree oil.

For wrinkles or aging skin, the best essential oils are the following: clary sage, frankincense, geranium, lavender, lemon, patchouli, rose, rosemary, sandalwood and ylang-ylang. Like with acne, choose your essential oil depending on your preferred scent, and if you have sensitive skin, depending on what does not give you irritation. You can also combine these oils to create a unique scent. Rose and patchouli will give you a sophisticated feminine scent while lavender and lemon will give a fresh and stimulating albeit still feminine scent.

You can apply these essential oils with your choice of carrier oil as described for acne. Since aging skin is usually dry, it is better to use olive, avocado or coconut oil. Argan and rosehip oils are more expensive options but they have additional anti-aging properties.

If you prefer a cream texture for your anti-aging skin care, you can also add shea butter or cocoa butter to your carrier oil. Use ¼ cup of shea or cocoa butter with

¼ cup of your choice of carrier oil, then add 10 to 20 drops of your choice of essential oil or a combination. Melt this over a low fire, stir well then pour into a sterilized glass jar. Allow to cool before putting the lid on. Keep this jar in a cool, dark place. If you live in a hot climate or if it is currently the summer months, keep this jar in the refrigerator.

Alternatively, coconut oil by itself can become solid depending on the temperature. You can whip ½ cup of solid coconut oil before adding 10 to 20 drops of essential oil. Stir well. Keep this in a clean jar in the refrigerator so it will not liquefy.

Acne and wrinkles can also benefit from a toner and steam facial using the same essential oils recommended for each problem. To make toner, use distilled water and a sterilized bottle. For every cup of water, add 10 to 15 drops of essential oil. You can also replace the water with strongly brewed tea to add some antioxidant benefits. For acne and for oily skins, you can use commercially available witch hazel solution. Dry skins can use rose water.

A toner can be used to provide extra cleansing or to refresh the face in the middle of the day. If you wish to do the latter, store your toner in a spray bottle. Allow the toner to dry on your face.

To make a steam facial, heat about 5 cups of water then place in a large bowl. Add 5 drops of essential oil then bend over the bowl with a towel over your face. Inhale deeply to obtain the most benefits. For acne, the steam will open your pores and clean the gunk out of them. For wrinkles, the steam will soften your skin and allow it to absorb your moisturizer better. Do this steam facial at least twice a week.

For fungal infections, tea tree oil and neem oil are the best choices. Use them pure to cure your ailment fast or dilute them with a very small amount of carrier oil if you find the scent too strong. You can also apply the essential oil on a cotton pad and use a bandage to keep it in place. To make the scent more appealing, add peppermint oil which can also help alleviate the itch. Also, use coconut oil as your carrier oil since it contains anti-fungal properties.

If your fungal infection is on the foot or hand, you can make a warm soak with essential oils. Pour hot (but not boiling) water onto a basin and add 10 to 20 drops of your chosen essential oil. Carefully lower your hand or foot onto the basin (make sure the water is not boiling hot or else you might burn yourself). Let it sit there until the water cools. Make sure that the infected area is fully submerged. If possible, do this every day before applying more essential oil to the area.

Psoriasis and eczema can be 'cured' the same way as fungal infections. I say 'cured' because these skin ailments are actually auto-immune diseases. They come and go depending on what happens to the whole body. Thus, essential oil 'cures' only alleviate the symptoms like dryness and itch. They can also help prevent infections when the skin is broken after inadvertently scratching too much.

In addition to tea tree oil and neem oil, psoriasis and eczema can be 'cured' with patchouli and peppermint oil.

For minor skin burns and wounds, essential oils can also help to make them heal faster. Take note that we are only talking about *minor* burns and wounds like sun burn and small cuts and grazes. More serious cases should be treated by medical professionals.

The best essential oils for burns are chamomile, lavender, marjoram, peppermint and tea tree oil. Combine 10 to 20 drops with ½ cup of pure aloe vera gel which has been proven to help promote healing or use them with your choice of carrier oil.

Before any treatment, ensure that the area is clean and free from any topical skin formulas like lotions which may interfere with your treatment. Apply your essential oil as often as possible.

For wounds, tea tree, oregano, and thyme oils are good for disinfecting. Apply the essential oil directly on the wound. For already infected wounds, you can use tea tree or lavender oil. After the wound has healed, you can use rose essential oil to help prevent scarring or to make the scar disappear faster.

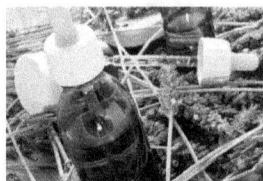

Chapter 3 – Hair Care

Essential oils can also be used to promote great hair. You can encourage faster hair growth, prevent hair damage and prevent frizz. There are also essential oils which can kill head lice and remove scalp psoriasis and dandruff.

For hair growth, rosemary or lavender essential oils are considered the best. Geranium, thyme, sage and ylang-ylang are also good choices. Combine them with your favorite commercial shampoo or apply them directly to the scalp with your favorite carrier oil. The latter will give you better results since you do not rinse off the essential oil. Also, your carrier oil will moisturize your hair and help to prevent frizz. Massage the essential oil with carrier oil onto your scalp for 10 minutes after shampooing. Leave this in your hair for the rest of the day like a conditioning hair oil, or you can do this at night if you dislike putting products on your hair.

For dry hair, use lavender, rosemary or geranium essential oils and combine them with the more emollient carrier oils like olive, coconut, avocado or argan oil. For a deep conditioning treatment, heat this combination until slightly warm then saturate the hair and scalp. Wrap the hair with towels wrung from hot water and leave it for at least an hour. You need to shampoo twice to get all the excess oils out. Do this at least once a month or once a week for best results. Use this same combination daily as a hair oil to prevent frizz.

For head lice, you can choose any of these essential oils: eucalyptus, lemon, thyme, rosemary, tea tree or geranium. Use 1:1 ratio of essential oil with your choice of carrier oil and apply all over the hair and scalp. Leave this for at least half an hour then shampoo it out. Do this until all the lice have died. The length of your treatment will depend on the population of lice on your head.

For scalp psoriasis, use the same recommendations for skin psoriasis but use a lighter carrier oil if you have oily hair.

Lastly, for dandruff, the best essential oils are tea tree oil and eucalyptus. You can use the same method described above for hair growth, but for your carrier oil use coconut oil. This oil has anti-fungal properties which will help kill the fungus which causes dandruff.

Chapter 4 – Carrier Oils

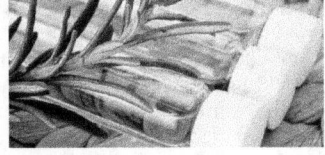

In this chapter, we will discuss carrier oils per se or which carrier oil is best for each specific ailment. If you can pair the best carrier oil with the best essential oil for your problems, then you will be able to solve your problem faster.

Carrier oils can be categorized either according to the skin or hair type they are fit for or according to the added advantages they can give like anti-fungal or anti-bacterial properties. Let us start with the first way of categorizing oils.

When we speak of skin or hair type, we talk of dry, normal or oily types. Dry skin is characterized by a lack of sebum or the oil which our skin naturally produces. This sebum is necessary to moisturize the skin and protect it from the elements like too much sun, wind and cold. Those with dry skin find that they easily form fine lines and wrinkles while those with oily skin often look younger during their middle age assuming they do not abuse their bodies with unhealthy habits. Granted that sebum alone is not enough to protect the skin from prolonged exposure to the elements, it at least provides *some* protection. Consider how those with dry skin easily burn from too much sun exposure or easily get itchy after being out too long during a windy or cold day. Dry skin is characterized by tightness and itchiness especially after washing the face with a non-moisturizing cleanser or during cold weather. It can even have tiny, dry flakes of skin hanging on the surface. This skin type is seldom plagued by pimples.

On the other hand, oily skin produces too much sebum. It can look shiny by the middle of the day or even earlier during hot weather when the oil glands are more active. While those with oily skin can look younger even during their older years because their skin is always moisturized, they can be plagued by pimples during their younger years.

Normal skin is considered balanced skin or what the skin should be. It is the ideal skin type and usually does not experience any problems except those which are caused by unhealthy habits like smoking, too much exposure to environmental pollution and an unhealthy diet. If normal skin is well taken care of, it will remain young-looking even until after middle-age.

Unfortunately for us, normal skin is very rare. It is more common for people to have combination skin which means that some areas like the forehead, nose and chin are oilier while the cheek areas are drier.

To check which skin type you have, you need to do this experiment: Wash your face with 10 splashes of water. You need to use water because your choice of cleanser might affect your results. A moisturizing cleanser will add moisture while a cleanser for oily skin might unnecessarily strip your skin. Dry your face with a towel but do not use anything, even toner. If your skin becomes oily all over, i.e. in all parts of your face, after 3 hours or less, you have very oily skin. If your skin becomes oily all over after 6 hours, you have oily skin. If it becomes oily after 8 hours, you have normal skin. If it becomes oily after more than 8 hours, you have normal to dry skin, i.e. dry skin that leans towards being normal. If it does not become oily at all, you have dry skin. If different parts of your face become oily at different times, then use the same criterion described above for those particular parts. Hence it is possible to have a very oily forehead but dry cheeks, and so on.

Take note that I have included the skin types 'very oily' and 'normal to dry.' This is because skin typing is actually better described like a spectrum. Some people will have an oily face after 4 or 5 hours, and some may even become shiny after only 2 hours. Also, your skin type can be affected by the climate you live in. Hot temperatures make the oil glands more active which is why those with normal skin can become oily during summer and dry during winter.

Also, skin type can change depending on your lifestyle choices and age. The skin becomes 10% drier every decade after the age of 20, so a teenager with very oily skin can expect some relief with age. It has also been proven that consuming too much processed foods and animal meats can make the skin oilier while smoking and too much alcohol can make the skin drier. Certain medications can also affect the skin type. In fact, birth control pills have been used by women to control their oil glands in order to keep their acne under control. Topical medications can also be used to control sebum production to help with acne problems.

Meanwhile, when we speak of dry, normal or oily hair, we are actually not 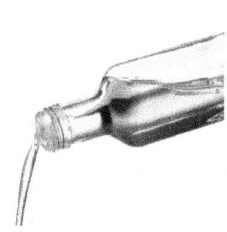 speaking of the hair but of the scalp. Hair is also moisturized and protected by sebum which is produced by the scalp. Sebum travels down the hair shaft either naturally or aided by frequent brushing. Dry hair is frizzy and easily tangled because the scalp produces little sebum while oily hair is lank and greasy because there is too much sebum. Normal hair will have a scalp that produces just enough sebum. As with skin, the hair can have very oily and normal to dry types too. The only difference is we do not have combination hair which will mean that some parts of the scalp are oilier than others. While it is possible to have this kind of scalp, it is difficult to check since the oils produced by some parts of the scalp easily spreads to other parts given that the hair strands are very close to each other. Also, as with the skin, the hair type can change with lifestyle and age. Since the scalp is also skin, it will be affected by one's diet and habits. Also, the scalp becomes drier with age which is why old people tend to have brittle hair.

To check which hair type you have, do the same experiment described above for the face, but instead of washing the hair with just water, wash it with a non-conditioning shampoo or a basic shampoo which adds no moisturizers, shine enhancing ingredients or anything else. A good example of this is basic, baby shampoo or mild soap. Rinse the hair well and do not add any hair products. If your hair roots become oily by the end of the day, you have oily hair. If they become oily after 2 days of not washing, you have normal hair. If they never become oily even if you have not washed it for 3 days, you have dry hair.

You need to wait a day or more to check which hair type you have because you cannot easily check your scalp unlike your hair. Also, the sebum produced by your scalp is immediately absorbed by your hair so it will not be easy to know how much sebum it produces.

It is a mistake to think that you will have the same skin and hair type. If it is possible to have combination skin, it is also possible to have a different type for the scalp. Thus, you can have dry hair and oily skin, and vice versa. If so, you might need to use different carrier oils for your face and hair.

If you have dry skin, the best carrier oils are those which are considered the most emollient. We have mentioned olive, rose hip, coconut and avocado oil in the previous chapters. Argan oil is also a very moisturizing albeit expensive option.

We have mentioned the use of cocoa butter and shea butter instead of carrier oils for a creamier texture. These are carrier substances but they also act like carrier oils in which they 'carry' and dilute the essential oil. Cocoa and shea butter are great options for dry skin, but shea is generally considered more emollient.

When buying butters, you have to make sure that they are not rancid. The best way to do this is to buy from reputable sources which label the date when these butters were made. Also, it is best to buy only the smallest amount possible and to keep it in the refrigerator. You should never use rancid butters especially if you have sensitive skin. Besides the possibility of irritation, they smell bad too. If your butter smells sour or unpleasant, throw it out. Fresh cocoa butter should smell like chocolate while shea should smell sweet and a little bit nutty.

You can also use coconut oil as a 'butter.' In cold temperatures, coconut oil solidifies which make it look like a butter. You can whip this to make it soft then keep your 'butter' in the refrigerator to prevent it from becoming liquid. If you live in colder climates or if summer has passed, your coconut oil 'butter' will likely remain solid even if it is not kept in the refrigerator.

For normal skin, you can use sweet almond, apricot kernel, jojoba or castor oil. The first two will give you a pleasant scent, while the last two will not have much of a scent. Jojoba is considered to be the closest in composition to sebum while castor oil has regenerative, anti-bacterial and anti-fungal properties. We will discuss more on this later.

If you prefer a cream consistency, instead of cocoa or shea butter, you can use beeswax. Though technically beeswax is not a butter but a wax, when mixed with an equal amount of one of the carrier oils listed above, the result is similar to a butter consistency but it is less emollient. This combination is perfect for normal skins.

Using beeswax is slightly more complicated than butters because you always have to melt the wax or else you will not be able to mix it with the other ingredients. Do not use pure beeswax with your essential oils or you will end up with a candle once the wax hardens.

For oily skin, the only carrier oil you must use is grape seed oil. This is the lightest of all the carrier oils. It also has an astringent effect, i.e. it can make the skin drier. As impossible as that sounds considering that we are talking about an oil, those with dry skins who have used grape seed oil report that they ended up with drier skins than they started with. This is because grape seed oil penetrates deeply into the skin and influences the oil glands to produce less sebum. It acts more like a serum rather than as an oil.

It is necessary to group the carrier oils or butters according to skin type first so you can limit your choices accordingly. After this, you can further limit your choice according to your further concerns.

Let us now discuss which oils are best for each specific concern.

For dry skin:

Fine lines and wrinkles

While all the oils listed above can be good for this problem because they are all very moisturizing, moisturizing the skin per se can be considered only a temporary solution to the signs of aging. What happens is the skin is temporarily plumped up so the fine lines and wrinkles become less obvious. However, if you really wish to diminish their appearance, here are your options starting from the best:

Rose hip oil – this oil contains vitamin C and A which are great antioxidants for the skin. Vitamin A encourages the skin to produce more collagen deep in the

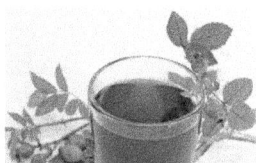

dermis resulting in smoother skin. It also gently exfoliates the skin resulting in a more radiant complexion. Vitamin C can also minimize dark spots.

Argan oil – this oil is very high in vitamin E which is an excellent antioxidant for turning back the clock.

Avocado – this oil contains anti-inflammatory

compounds called sterolins which help heal sun damage and age spots. If you are relatively young but see signs of skin damage, this might be a good choice for you to minimize premature aging.

Olive or coconut (your choice depending on your scent preference) – these oils are very emollient, but they have less anti-aging compounds compared to the above oils.

What about shea and cocoa butters? These are very good for moisturizing dry skin, but they are primarily used to make your natural skin care products more like a cream than a liquid oil. You must add other ingredients for additional benefits.

Dark spots

Rose hip oil is the best choice. (See above for the explanation.) Avocado oil can work for younger skins.

Fungal infections and dandruff

Coconut oil is best since it has natural anti-fungal properties. In fact, if you have used up your tea tree or lavender oil, you can just use coconut oil for fungal infections. It will take longer to heal without the essential oil, but all the same this proves how effective coconut oil is.

Eczema and psoriasis

As we have discussed, essential oils and carrier oils can only alleviate symptoms, not completely cure these ailments. Either olive or coconut oils are good choices to minimize the dryness of eczema and psoriasis.

Acne

If you have dry skin and acne, the best combination is coconut oil and tea tree, lavender or neem oil. Coconut oil has natural anti-bacterial properties which will keep inflammation at bay. You can alternate coconut oil with rose hip oil. The vitamin A in rose hip will help to exfoliate the skin of dead skin cells (one of the causes of acne) and will keep acne scars to a minimum.

For normal skin:

Fine lines and wrinkles

The oils fit for normal skin generally do not work well for minimizing fine lines and wrinkles, but they are good for preventing them.

Jojoba, sweet almond and apricot kernel oils can prevent fine lines and wrinkles only by moisturizing the skin. As discussed above, skin that is moisturized is well protected from the elements. These oils can replace sebum especially during the times when the skin produces less sebum like during the colder months.

You can also use these oils to lighten, i.e. make less emollient, the oils for dry skins to obtain their benefits.

What about beeswax? Beeswax is like cocoa or shea butter for dry skin. It is used to make a cream consistency, but it will not give you other benefits.

Dark spots

Castor oil can help heal dark spots given its healing abilities. However, it will work slower compared to rose hip oil. You can combine the two to lighten rose hip oil and to make your dark spots disappear faster.

Fungal infections and dandruff

Castor oil is the best choice for this problem because it contains the compound undecylenic acid which has anti-fungal properties.

Eczema and psoriasis

For alleviating dryness, jojoba, sweet almond or apricot kernel oil are good choices.

Acne

Castor oil contains anti-bacterial properties from ricinoleic acid. It will be less effective than coconut oil, but since it is lighter than the former, it can be a better choice for normal skin types.

For oily skin:

Oily skins can only use grape seed oil because using any other oil will result to excess greasiness. Fortunately, grape seed oil has a variety of benefits. It can help to regenerate the skin and minimize the signs of aging, alleviate the dryness of eczema and psoriasis and can help acne issues by making the oil glands produce less oil. However, it cannot help with fungal infections unless you use it with an essential oil like tea tree oil or lavender.

For hair issues:

Dry hair

Use the carrier oils prescribed for dry skin. However, avoid using the butters since they can leave a waxy film on the hair which can be difficult to remove.

Hair growth

Use castor oil as your carrier oil since this is proven to encourage hair to grow longer. You can also use pure castor oil to encourage eye lashes to grow longer. How long your lashes will grow still depends on your genetic make-up. Those who have naturally long lashes will still end up with longer lashes than those who have naturally short ones, but the point here is you will see an improvement. Also, you can use castor oil to encourage your brows to grow. This is particularly helpful if you accidentally shaved or plucked too much.

If you wish to try using castor oil on brows or lashes, Use a cotton bud to apply the castor oil and do not double dip into the bottle to avoid the spread of bacteria. Some people use their clean fingertip, but it is still more hygienic to use a clean cotton bud. Double dipping or using dirty tools can lead to eye infection especially for the lashes. You have to apply the castor oil on the eyelash roots, not on the eye lashes themselves. Do this carefully to avoid poking your eye, but don't be afraid if you get some oil on your eye. This will not be painful or hurt you in the long run; however, if you use contact lenses, remove them first before applying the oil. Also, don't re-insert your contact lenses. It is better to do this at night before sleeping so you don't have to use contact lenses anymore. To remove excess oil, pat tissue over your closed eye. You can expect to see results in 4 to 8 weeks assuming you do this at least once every day. To speed up things, you can apply castor oil at least 3 times throughout the day.

Do not add essential oil to the castor oil if you wish to use it on your lashes. Doing this can lead to irritation since it is an area which is very near the eye ball. You can use essential oil for the eye brows but just make sure that none gets into the eye. Sensitive eyes or eyes which easily tear up must avoid the essential oil especially lavender whose irritating fumes can reach the eye from the brows.

Castor oil was recommended for minimizing the signs of skin aging, but if it can also be used to encourage hair growth, will you end up with a beard? It sounds funny, but you don't have to worry about this. Castor oil only encourages hair growth but it does not create new hair follicles in the skin. It is true that a woman's facial skin is covered with tiny hairs, but these hair follicles can only grow short, tiny hairs. Even if castor oil encourages them to grow, they will only grow exactly what they are already growing: short, tiny, almost invisible hairs. It would be a different situation for a man whose facial hair follicles grow thick hair much like the head. Castor oil can help him to grow a longer beard should he wish to do so.

Lice

Removing lice will be easier if you use coconut oil as your carrier oil. It will drown the lice and dissolve the glue which adheres nits to the hair shaft.

Scalp psoriasis and dandruff

For scalp psoriasis, you can use any carrier oil which will help to dissolve the scales and alleviate dry, itchy skin.

As already mentioned above, coconut oil is good for dandruff which is caused by excess fungi on the scalp.

Chapter 5– Stress and Pain Relief

Another use for essential oils is to relieve stress and some minor aches and pains. For stress relief, usually essential oils are inhaled through oil burners or diffusers, dry evaporation, room sprays or steam inhalation. Oil burners are ceramic containers with a shallow bowl on top and space for a tea light underneath. The essential oil is placed on the shallow bowl, an equal amount of water is added and the tea light warms the solution to diffuse the scent. Essential oils should never be directly heated because this will change their scent. There are also electric appliances called diffusers which work on the same principle of warming the essential oil to release its scent. Alternatively, scented candles can be used.

For safety reasons, never leave an oil burner, diffuser or candle alone for several hours to avoid overheating. This can also change the scent of your essential oil.

For dry evaporation, the essential oil is applied to cotton, tissues or potpourri and the scent is allowed to disperse. This method will give a more subtle scent. You can also scent handkerchiefs and pillow cases. Room sprays work like body perfume. The essential oils are mixed with alcohol or water then this solution is sprayed to scent the room.

Lastly, steam inhalation works by inhaling the steam from hot water mixed with a few drops of essential oil like the steam facial described above. The last method is very potent because the nose is directly over the hot water. Only 1 to 2 drops of essential oils must be used or else the scent can be too overwhelming.

The method you choose will depend on your personal preferences. For example, while steam inhalation is the most potent, this can be too tedious for some. Busy people might find that room sprays or dry evaporation are more convenient.

As for the essential oil to choose, here are some options depending on your specific concern:

Anxiety – lavender, geranium, orange, patchouli

Depression – chamomile, jasmine, bergamot, rose

Insomnia – lavender, chamomile

To increase energy or to stimulate the mind – peppermint, rosemary, lemon, vanilla, grapefruit

An even more convenient way to decrease stress is to use essential oils as a perfume. If you are going to do this, make sure that you use true essential oils and not fragrance oils since you will apply this directly to your skin. Also, with the former the scent will be superior in quality.

Essential Oils Box Set #33: Essential Oils & Aromatherapy for Beginners & The Beginners Guide to Medicinal Plants

You need to use carrier oils since directly applying essential oil to your skin will result in a too strong scent. Use half an ounce of neutral smelling vegetable oil like grape seed or sunflower oil then add the recommended amount of essential oils.

Here are some recipes for your stress-busting perfume:

Feminine	• 2 drops vanilla and 3 drops lavender
Citrus	• Equal amounts of lemon, grapefruit, and orange
Spicy	• 5 drops patchouli, 1 drop cinnamon

These are only recommended recipes but feel free to experiment to get your desired scent. When it comes to perfume, though the above are supposed to be for reducing stress, you still want to smell good. Allow the scent to combine with your own natural scent to see if it results in a pleasant fragrance. You might need to ask someone else to judge the resulting combination. It might take some time before you find the best recipe for yourself, but the above recipes are good starting points. The above combinations can also be used for your oil burner or room spray.

If you are going to use essential oils for pain relief like headaches and muscle pains, direct application to the painful area will be more effective. Peppermint, lavender and rosemary are the best choices for headaches. You can use the pure essential oil or combine it with carrier oil if you find the scent to be too strong. Apply a drop of this on the area of your head which feels painful. Take note that if you need to apply the essential oil on your temple or forehead, you might irritate your eyes. If so, you need to use a drop of carrier oil. Alternatively, you might wish to close your eyes and lie back for a while to hasten your healing.

For muscle aches, essential oils help to increase circulation and warm the muscle to sooth it. The best essential oils for general muscle pains include the following: basil, rosemary, clary sage, chamomile, lavender and elemi.

Sometimes, your muscle pains may be accompanied by inflammation. Examples of this situation include muscle strains or sprains. For these cases, essential oils which help reduce inflammation are better choices. These include: peppermint, lavender, clove, thyme and marjoram.

Lastly, essential oils can also help relax the muscles after a long day at work. The best way to relax the muscle is through massage. Combine 5 to 10 drops of the following essential oils with 1 cup of unscented massage oil: rosemary, peppermint, ginger, eucalyptus.

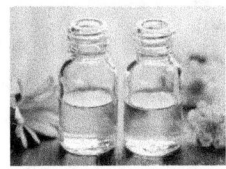 # Chapter 6 – Weight Loss

Through aromatherapy, essential oils can also help boost your mood while you are trying to lose weight. Take note that the weight loss effect here is only indirect, more like a motivational speech than something which will actually make you burn excess calories. You cannot realistically expect essential oils to replace exercise and a healthy diet.

When using essential oils for weight loss, you can internally ingest 1 to 2 drops combined with a glass of water, tea or other liquid throughout the day or you can also sniff the scent. Do both these methods for the best results.

To be on the safe side, start with 1 drop and see if you experience any uncomfortable sensations or digestive problems. If 1 week has passed and you do not experience anything bad, move on to 2 drops. However, if you suddenly experience something bad, move back to 1 drop and stick with that amount.

Regarding the ingestion of essential oils, make sure that you are using true essential oils and not fragrance oils. The latter might be poisonous. Also, not all essential oils can be ingested. For example, tea tree oil is particularly dangerous and even a small amount can prove fatal if taken internally.

Make sure you are ingesting high quality essential oils which do not contain any impurities. The label should say 100% essential oil, and it should say that it has been tested for purity. This is an important precaution because impure essential oils can contain poisonous substances. This is also why you must start with using just 1 drop when trying this. If you wish to be even more cautious, ingest the drop of essential oil only every other day so you can observe the effect on your body. However, all the same, it is still best to ensure that the brand of essential oil you choose is pure and safe.

Those which are safe to ingest for weight loss include the following: grapefruit, lemon, peppermint and ginger. Take note that these essential oils are commonly used for cooking. To further ensure that you are ingesting safe essential oils, buy them from cooking supply stores rather than from your general essential oil store.

For variety, you can choose to cook with these essential oils (after you have checked for their safety). Add them to salad dressings, marinades or baked goods. Use a proportion which will ensure that the finished dish provides only 1 or 2 drops of essential oil per serving. For example, if the recipe provides 5 servings, add at most only 10 drops of essential oil.

Here are some further ideas:

- Add your choice of essential oil to your cake or muffin recipes. However, make sure that you avoid frosting the cake with high calorie frosting or whipped cream since you don't want to cancel out your weight loss efforts. You can also use no-calorie sweetener instead of sugar to further lessen the calories.

- Add a few drops of grapefruit or lemon essential oil to sauces to be served with fish.

- Mix 5 drops of lemon essential oil with 100 ml soy sauce. This will give the soy sauce a lemony aroma. It can be used as a dip for fish, sushi and for other uses where soy sauce is called for.

- Instead of lemon juice, use lemon essential oil. Use 4 drops to replace the juice from a medium lemon. Do the same for recipes calling for grapefruit juice, but use 6 drops since grapefruits are bigger. Make up for the lesser liquid by adding water. For ginger, use 1 drop for every inch square of ginger called for.

- Add a few drops of peppermint essential oil to your marinade for lamb. Lamb and mint are a classic combination.

- Add 3 drops of peppermint essential oil to non-fat whipped topping. This can be used as a minty topping for sugar-free hot chocolate or coffee. Alternatively, you can add 1 drop of peppermint to hot chocolate or coffee. This is a great drink for the winter holidays. Just ensure that you use no-calorie sweetener.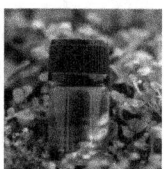

- Add 1 drop of peppermint essential oil to a cup of fruit salad for a refreshing zing which is especially good during the summer months. Don't add any sweetener.

- Add peppermint or ginger essential oil to lemonade or other summer drinks.

- Add ginger essential oil and ginger bread spices like cinnamon and nutmeg to your pancake or other quick bread recipes to give it a gingerbread twist.

- Add your choice of essential oil to sugar-free gelatin for a quick snack that helps with your weight loss.

- Use a few drops of your choice of essential oil to flavor merengue. A 1-inch merengue cookie, even if sugar is used, only provides 15 calories making it a great choice for times when you get a sugar craving.

Here are ideas for sniffing these essential oils to aid weight loss:

- Use an oil burner, diffuser or candle while exercising and during meals. Using room sprays require you to keep spraying while potpourri might not give a strong enough scent for your purposes.

- Sniff your choice of essential oil before every meal to help you control your appetite.

- Once you finish your food, sniff the essential oil again to avoid going back for seconds.

- If you are plagued by emotional eating, e.g. eating when stressed even if you are not hungry, sniff your essential oil.

Regularly ingesting these essential oils or regularly sniffing them can help to suppress your appetite and keep your metabolism under control. Again, take note that the operative word here is 'help.' You still have to continue with your usual reduced calorie diet and regular exercise regime.

Chapter 7 – Caution When Using Essential Oils

In this chapter, we will discuss some precautions you need to take when using essential oils. In the previous chapter, I assumed that you do not suffer from any health condition or are not pregnant. Also, I assume that you are an adult. Otherwise, there are certain precautions.

First, you need to make sure that you are not allergic to the essential oil or the carrier oils or butters you choose to use. Generally speaking, if you have a food allergy to a substance, you will also have a topical allergy to it. For example, if you are allergic to nuts, you will probably also get an allergic reaction when you apply shea butter (which comes from a nut) on your skin. There are cases where having a food allergy does not mean having a skin allergy, but you should be better safe than sorry. After all, you have a variety of other options besides shea butter.

Still regarding allergies, most people who do not have a lot of allergies will probably not be allergic to any of the essential oils listed in this book. However, if you have a lot of allergies, food or skin, then it is best to do a skin test before using an essential oil or a carrier oil or butter.

To do a skin test, get a small amount of the ingredients you wish to use. Apply a small amount on a hidden part of your body like the inside of the elbow, under the knee or behind the ear. Leave the substance for at least 24 hours. If irritation occurs, wash off the substance and apply some medicated cream which will help with the irritation. You must not use that substance in the future. Make sure that you test each substance individually otherwise you will not be able to know which caused the allergy, the essential oil or carrier oil.

Second, essential oils must be stored away from children and pets. They can be curious about these oils and inadvertently cause harm to themselves or others. Take note too that essential oils are flammable. If you are using them for aromatherapy, make sure that your oil burner or diffuser is safe. Low quality oil burners can allow the essential oil and water mixture to seep through the ceramic bowl and drip on the candle thus causing the flame to become bigger. If your oil burner is placed near curtains or furniture, it can result to a bigger fire.

Third, if you encounter an unfamiliar essential oil, do your research first to make sure you will not hurt yourself. It is best to stick to the tried and tested oils. Why should you try out an unfamiliar essential oil if you know that what you are currently using is working? Some can also be toxic like wormwood which can result in hallucinations and pennyroyal which can cause miscarriage, organ damage and even death. These names are usually unfamiliar to many people, but just in case you encounter them in the store, make sure you avoid them.

Reputable stores will likely not sell these to people, but some stores might carry them for experienced users of these essential oils.

Fourth, always start with the smallest recommended dose when trying out an essential oil even if they are already familiar like lavender. This is just to avoid unforeseen complications. Once you are sure that you will experience no irritation or discomfort, you can progress to the higher amounts.

Fifth, it is best to avoid using essential oils for newborns and very young infants. They still have very sensitive skins which may be irritated if applied with essential oils. If you need something for certain problems like eczema, it is better to use coconut oil which is proven to be gentle enough for baby's skin. Apricot kernel oil is also a good choice for young skin. At any rate, very young children are usually still not plagued by the issues discussed here.

Sixth, do not assume that all essential oils can be used for aromatherapy. Some essential oils like neem smell bad and may make you nauseous.

Seventh, pregnant and nursing women must be careful when using essential oils. Many are not safe for them even if they are used for skin conditions or fragrance because they can be absorbed by the skin and brought into the bloodstream or milk glands where they will eventually affect the fetus or infant. Here are the essential oils which pregnant women can safely use: rose, chamomile, jasmine, lavender, geranium, sandalwood, frankincense. Generally speaking, pregnant women should not ingest essential oils for whatever reason until they have given birth.

You might ask: even perfume is not allowed? Cologne or eau de toilette which contains only a very small percentage of essential oil compared to alcohol is safe. What I am referring to above is the pure essential oil. You can try using it with diluted with carrier oil, but why would you risk your health and your baby's?

Eighth, those who suffer from certain medical conditions **should avoid** certain essential oils used in any way, including aromatherapy:

Epilepsy – rosemary, sage, camphor and fennel (These can encourage seizures.)

High blood pressure – rosemary, sage, thyme

Asthma – marjoram

Hepatitis or cirrhosis – avoid **all** essential oils

Ninth, certain essential oils must not be used in the *long term* or else they can be toxic due to a build-up of harmful toxins in the body. These include cinnamon, juniper, coriander, eucalyptus, turmeric and laurel.

Tenth, if you will be exposed to the sun, avoid using these oils since they can cause dark spots to form: bergamot, cedar wood, ginger, grapefruit, and patchouli. If you use any of these for skin care or other purposes, use them at night or else on an area that is not touched by sun light.

Eleventh, take note of the scent and appearance of the essential oil when fresh. If they change scent, color and viscosity, toss them. Citrus essential oils usually last for only a year while flowers last for up to 5 years if they are stored properly. Those with the heavier scents like sandalwood, patchouli and frankincense can last up to several years.

This is the reason why essential oils are usually sold in small bottles. Since they are concentrated, you only need to use a small amount. Keeping a large bottle, unless you have many uses for it, will only result in waste.

Twelfth, if you are in doubt, don't. If you need to do more research, do so. It is important to understand that essential oils are medicines. Even if they are not regulated in the same way as prescription medication, they can still cause harm if misused. If you need further advice on how to use certain essential oils, go beyond books and internet sources by consulting an actual expert. Just like how you need to go to an actual doctor if your sickness is serious instead of just depending on books or internet sources, a direct discussion with an essential oil expert will allow you to voice out all your concerns. It will also allow the expert to judge which essential oil is best for your specific situation after considering all relevant information like allergies, past and present medical conditions and personal preferences.

Conclusion

Thank you again for purchasing this book!

I hope this book was able to help you to use essential oils for your various ailments.

The next step is to try out the tips for yourself and experiment to know what works for you. As long as you are careful and always test your new concoctions, you can be sure that essential oils will only give you many benefits.

Finally, if you enjoyed this book, please take the time to share your thoughts and post a review on Amazon. We do our best to reach out to readers and provide the best value we can. Your positive review will help us achieve that. It'd be greatly appreciated!

Thank you and good luck!

Book 2

The Beginners Guide to Medicinal Plants

BY LINDSEY P

Everything You Need to Know About the Healing Properties of Plants & Herbs, How to Grow and Harvest Them

Table Of Contents

Introduction

I want to thank you and congratulate you for purchasing the book, *"The Beginners Guide to Medicinal Plants"*.

This book contains proven steps and strategies on how to successfully grow medicinal plants and herbs right at the very comfort of your own home.

Featured in this book are some of the most common mistakes when putting up a medicinal garden at home and how to avoid committing such mistakes. Also featured in this book are some of the best types of medicinal plants to grow at home.

Thanks again for purchasing this book, I hope you enjoy it!

Chapter 1: Guide to Growing a Medicinal Herb Garden

Growing medicinal plants and herbs indoor is a popular hobby for a lot of gardeners. One of the greatest reasons to plant medicinal plants indoor is to have a ready supply of these beneficial herbs. These herbs are those that you commonly snip into your sauces and soups. They can also be used to soothe an itchy rash or cough. Growing medicinal herbs may not sound to be very appealing, however you can benefit from growing these plants that can provide instant relief for many illnesses that can happen anytime of the day.

It would also be wonderful to be able to cut a sprig of thyme while boiling water and prepare a fresh cup of thyme tea that is fragrant and vibrant. Since it is fresh, you'll sure it is effective since it's fresh.

So what kind of medicinal plants should you grow? The next chapter of this book features a list of different herbs and medicinal plants that you can grow at home. The list is just a good starting point for easy to find and easy to grow herbs. The same plants that you can use in cooking daily may also be used as teas, salves, washes and tinctures. You can also make cough syrup and cough drops with the very same herbal plants that you grow in the comforts of your own home.

No matter how you thoroughly care for your medicinal plants, in the long run, they will have to be replaced. If this should happen during the colder days, you will have to take into account the growing time, before they will be big enough for harvest. Commonly, this will take about 4 to 6 weeks. You can make use of these herbs not only for cooking but for medicinal purposes as well.

What problems can you possibly encounter while growing medicinal plants and herbs in your home garden? While herbs typically suffer from much less issues that flowers and vegetables do, there are a few things that should be looked out for. Plants grown in your home garden may also encounter some basic problems such as molds or mildew problems, insect damage and most of all, fertilizer issues. To remedy these problems, you must know the following guidelines:

1. Home Garden Temperature

    While most of us think our homes as a temperate area would be ideal for growing plants, this is not always the case.

    A plant requires light in order to make food, a process which we know as photosynthesis. While plants are very adaptable, they grow best within a 70 to 75 degree range. A plant utilizes more energy when the temperature is warm than when it is cold. Plants can adapt to a cooler room, for instance, with an air conditioner. The plants will begin the process of photosynthesis with the increase in temperature and there will be no sunlight to produce food. When this happens, the plants will not most likely to thrive and will probably die.

So what is the best temperature for growing medicinal herbs?

Plants grow best when there is at least a 10 degree fall in temperature during the night. During the summer, the temperature tends to get high and stay high. Plants get stressed and become highly susceptible to diseases. They grow less and can drop leaves, weaken and die, despite sufficient watering. If you are growing herbs indoors, it would be a good idea to grow them around a room based on available temperature zones. Save a lot of money and be stress-free by working on with what you already have instead of trying to make big modifications that work against the natural rhythm of your home environment.

2. Home Garden Fertilizer

Once you have already decided on which type of herbs that you will grow in your home garden, you will now have to choose the most suitable fertilizer for them. Not all fertilizers are created the same. While most have advertising claims, these fertilizers may be overused enough to damage your medicinal herbs grown at home.

What kinds of fertilizers can be used at home? There are a lot of fertilizer types that will work for your medicinal herb garden at home. For indoor plants, you can try using a variety that can be dissolved in water (water-soluble). This particular type of fertilizer may come in packaged granular form that you measure and dissolve in water prior to application. It may also come in the form of a fish emulsion, which is a concentrated variety and is combined with water before application.

Regardless on the type of fertilizer that you choose to use, you must apply it at one quarter of the packaging's recommended amount. Apply this light mixture once every week. For a more effective application, make sure to water your plants thoroughly and then apply the prepared fertilizer solution. This technique will allow for better absorption by the plant.

More importantly, make sure that you do a monthly flushing of your medicinal plants. This can be done by placing the plant in a sink and water entirely, allowing the excess water to draw off. Once the dripping stops, water completely once again. This technique will get rid of any salts that may have accumulated in the plant's soil.

Chapter 2: Easy Guide to Successfully Grow Herbs and Medicinal Plants at Home

Follow this easy step-by-step guide to start with your medicinal herb garden at home:

1. Choose your herbs. When growing medicinal herbs at home, it is important to have a good variety of herbs as well as companion plants. Some of the good choice include the following:

   - Hot pepper

   - Strawberries

   - Oregano

   - Thyme

   - Lime basil

   - Mint

   - Common basil

   - Sage

   - Lemon balm

   - Sweet marjoram

2. Prepare your pot. Be sure that the pots that you will be using for your medicinal plants have holes at the bottom to provide good drainage. With a grit or gravel, pour to about a quarter of the pot's depth. This will allow the water to steep out from the soil's bottom.

3. Fill. When the gravel is already in place, begin to fill the pot with soil-based or multi-purpose compost. Fill t about three (3) quarters of the pot's remaining space.

4. Begin planting – put the medicinal plants into the pot, with around 15 centimeters between each stem. Squeeze every plant lightly from its temporary pot. To encourage the plants to spread out, tease the roots from the root ball.

5. Put the trailing plants near the edge and the taller ones in the center of the display. This technique will endure the best growth for your plants. DO not worry if the display may seem to appear messy at first. This will begin to fill out and look lush in just a few weeks.

6. Fill in the spaces around the plants. When you are already satisfied with the positions, begin filling in the gaps in between the plants with compost. Tightly push the compost into the spaces by pushing your fingers deep into the soil. Be careful not to injure the roots. Add more if needed. To avoid overflowing when being waters, leave a few centimeters between the rim of the pot and the soil.

7. Top the plants. Cut the taller plants' top. This will encourage them to bush out and give more fresh leaves to pick during harvest time.

8. Fertilize regularly. Purchase a controlled release fertilizer which should last a whole season. This will mean that you won't have to feed the pot again.

9. Water. Water your plants thoroughly or until the water begins to drain out of the pot's bottom. Medicinal plants usually like to dry out between watering and some types of medicinal plants such as Rosemary can easily be over-watered.

Growing herbs and medicinal plants at home is an easy yet a very rewarding hobby. Below are seven (7) key steps that will surely help you to successfully grow a healthy medicinal herb at home:

1. Keep an eye on Pests

    Medicinal herbs are generally not bothered so much about pests as much as flowers and vegetables can be. In an indoor garden however, the non-natural conditions may increase the possibility of a pest problem. To keep pests from damaging your medicinal plants in your indoor garden, make sure to keep a close eye. At the very first sight of infestation, make use of a soapy spray. You may also handpick any pests that you may have come to notices and put sticky traps to get rid of the rest.

2. Water your plants regularly

    Medicinal herbs require thorough attention when it comes to watering. Whether your medicinal plants likes drier conditions or extra moisture, it is never a good idea to have plants to be sitting in water.

3. Apply fertilizer

    Always keep in mind that medicinal plants grown indoors require a special fertilization schedule than those which are planted in an outdoor environment.

4. Be mindful of the soil

Indoor gardening soil needs to have effective exceptional drainage. It also needs to be light. Whether your medicinal plants like drier conditions or with extra moisture, having your plants to sit in water is never a good idea. Specifically buy potting soil. You may also prepare your own by using a part of peat moss, a part of sand and a part of bagged potting soil.

5. Ensure proper circulation

Medicinal plants require sufficient airflow to keep pests and bacterial organisms at bay. Just make sure to keep the air moving in the area where you will grow your medicinal plants.

6. Check your temperature

Keep your planting area at constant temperature. The ideal temperature for a home garden is about 60 to 70 degrees.

7. Provide enough light

Provide about 14 to 16 hours of artificial light to keep your medicinal plants healthy. You can also alternatively expose them to natural light for about 6 hours a day.

Chapter 3: The Best Medicinal Plants to Grow at Home

Do you have a small space at home to grow some plants? Why not grow some medicinal plants? Growing your own medicinal plants will not only get a lot of enjoyment but this will also provide medicinal relief at the comforts of your own home. While herbal remedies must never take the place of professional health care, it would be nice to have a sense of self-help should you ever end up having to need instant relief. Below is a list of the best plants to start your own personal medicinal plants garden:

1. Echinacea – this herb is also popularly known as the purple coneflower. Echinacea is an American perennial wildflower which is popularly known for its stimulating effects in the immune system. Preparations made with this wonder herb are used for the treatment of flu, colds, minor infections and a wide range of various illnesses.

2. Lavender – is medicinal plant which is commonly used as a fragrance these days. Lavender has been widely used since ancient times to reduce swelling, provide relief for rashes and itching and to treat burns, bug bites and other skin orders.

3. Lemon Balm – Prepare potent lemonade by adding bruised lemon balm leaves into your drink. This herb is commonly used as a calming "night tea" to combat insomnia. It can also make an effective topical relief for cold sores.

4. Comfrey – The roots of this wonder herb are cooked and mashed to make a potent topical relief for sprains, burns, bruises and arthritis. Just do not eat it. There is a study which reported that this herb can potentially damage the liver in eaten in significant amounts.

5. St. John's Wort – this wonder herb can lift the mood very well that you must keep from using this when you are already taking other forms of anti-depressants. The flowers and leaves of this herb may be used to prepare a tea. They can also be soaked in liquor to make a tincture. In a recent announcement, the FDA warned the public that there was a risk of adverse reactions between this herb and certain prescription drugs used for the treatment of cancer, transplant rejection, heart disease and AIDS, among others.

6. Borage – this potent herb has beautiful flowers that may be soaked in alcohol to prepare a powerful tonic that can boost your mood. The flowers and leaves may be used in tea preparations, eaten raw or soaked in liquor or wine to flavor the drink. The fresh plant provides a salty flavor with a cucumber-like smell.

7. Peppermint – this medicinal plant can be an effective tonic to promote better digestion. However, peppermint and any other strong mints such as pennyroyal must not be taken by women who are pregnant or possibly be pregnant. Drinks and foods that have fresh strong mint leaf can be harmful to the baby.

8. Pennyroyal – just like peppermint, pennyroyal is a great smelling mint which can be crushed and topically applied to the skin as a very powerful insect repellent. The leaves of pennyroyal can be crushed and topically applied to wounds as an antiseptic agent. It can also be used in tea preparations to tame upset stomach, however, do not over do it. The maximum recommendation is 2 cups daily. Consuming more than this recommendation may cause cramps and nausea.

9. Aloe vera – is a plant native to tropical Africa. This plant has spread worldwide as a first medicinal herb that provides soothing effects for scalds and burns. Aloe vera is best grown in a container so that it can be easily transferred indoors during the winter season.

10. Yarrow – for someone who's about to start a medicinal garden at home, yarrow is usually the top pick. This herb is a beautiful perennial plant that can serve a lot of different uses. Crushed yarrow flowers and leaves may be directly applied to scratches and cuts to reduce the chances of infections and to stop bleeding.

11. Slippery Elm – the inner back of this wonder herb can be ground and made into a nutrient-rich porridge-like soup. This can be an effective remedy for sore throat. In addition to this, the inner bark of this herb can be soothe irritations in the digestive tract.

12. Fenugreek – the seeds of this medicinal plant are nourishing and used to:

- Restore a dull sense of taste

- Freshen the breath

- Ease labor pains

- Ease painful menstruation

- Help in insufficient lactation

- Promote better digestion

- Help for late onset diabetes

- Darin off sweat ducts

- Treat inflammation and ulcers of the intestines and stomach

- Reduce blood cholesterol levels

- Inhibit cancer of the liver

- Encourage weight gain

13. Feverfew – is a plant which can be made into tea for the treatment of fevers, colds and arthritis. This plant is said to have sedative properties. It can also regulate menstruation. A feverfew infusion may be used to bathe swollen feet. It can also be made into a tincture for the treatment of bruises. Chewing about 4 pieces of leaves daily has been proven to be an effective cure for some migraine headaches.

14. Comfrey – an herb which contains allantoin. This substance is a cell proliferant which boosts the natural replacement of body cells. Comfrey is widely known for its ability to build strong teeth and bones in children. Comfrey is safer to use externally than internally. This wonder herb is used to treat a wider variety of health issues including the following:

- Varicose veins

- Eczema

- Sores

- Sprains

- Bruises

- Cuts

- Acne

- Severe burns

- Varicose and gastric ulcers

- Arthritis

- Sprains

- Broken bones

- Bronchial problems

15. Milk Thistle – this powerful herb can protect and improve the function of the liver. This herb may be taken internally to help treat the following:

- The effects of a hangover

- The growth of cancer cells in prostate, cervical and breast cancer

- Insulin resistance in patients suffering from type 2 diabetes who also have cirrhosis

- Increased cholesterol levels

- Liver inflammation or hepatitis

- Jaundice

- Gall bladder diseases

- Liver diseases

16. Wu Wei Zi – the fruit of this herb are reported to stimulate the central nervous system when used in low doses. In large doses, the fruits are said to depress the central nervous system while regulating the cardiovascular system. The seeds of this herb are used in the treatment of cancer. When used externally, this herb is used to treat allergic and irritating skin problems. Internally, this herb is used to treat the following conditions:

- Diabetes

- Hepatitis

- Hyperacidity

- Poor memory

- Insomnia

- Palpitations

- Chronic diarrhea

- Involuntary ejaculation

- Urinary disorders

- Night sweats

- Asthma

- Dry coughs

17. Sage – the latin name for this herb, "salvia", means to heal. When used internally, this herb treats the following conditions:

- Menopausal problems

- Femal sterility

- Depression

- Anxiety

- Excessive salivation

- Excessive perspiration

- Excessive lactation

- Liver issues

- Flatulence

- Indigestion

When used externally, sage is used for:

- Vaginal discharge

- Skin infections

- Gum infections

- Mouth infections

- Throat infection

- Skin infections

- Insect bites

18. Turkey Rhubarb – this herb is popularly known for its beneficial and positive effect on the digestive system. Even children can take advantage of the beneficial effects of this herb because it is gentle enough. In low doses, the roots can serve as an astringent tonic for better digestion while higher doses may be used as laxatives. In addition to this, turkey rhubarb is also known to treat the following:

- Skin eruptions because of toxin accumulation

- Menstrual problems

- Hemorrhoids

- Gall bladder problems

- Liver diseases

- Diarrhea

- Chronic constipation

19. Ginseng – is one of the most highly repudiated medicinal herbs in the orient. This wonder herb is touted for its ability to promote overall health, and general body vigor. The roots of this amazing medicinal plant is used to:

- Treat insomnia

- Address lack of appetite

- Treat debility related to old age

- Boost resistance against diseases

- Reduce levels of cholesterol

- Reduce blood sugar levels

- Enhance stamina

- Promote secretion of hormones

- Relax and stimulate the nervous system

20. Evening Primrose - the young roots of this medicinal plant can be consumed like a vegetable. The shoots may also be eaten as a salad. The roots of this wonder herb can be applied to bruises and piles. The roots may also be made into tea for the treatment of bowel pains and obesity. However, the more valuable parts are the bark and the leaves which are made into evening primrose oil, which is popularly known to treat the following conditions:

- Alcohol-associated liver damage

- Rheumatoid arthritis

- Brittle nails

- Acne

- Eczema

- Hyperactivity

- Premenstrual tension

- Multiple sclerosis

21. Tea tree – even the aborigines have utilized the leaves of tea tree for medicinal purposes, such as chewing fresh leaves to ease headaches. The

twigs, and leaves are made into tea tree oil which has antiseptic, antibacterial and antifungal properties. Tea tree oil definitely deserves a place in every household medicine cabinet. Tea tree oil is widely used for the treatment of the following illnesses:

- Minor burns

- Nits

- Cold sores

- Insect bites

- Warts

- Athlete's foot

- Acne

- Vaginal infections

- Thrush

- Chronic fatigue syndrome

- Glandular fever

- Cystitis

22. Great yellow gentian – the root of this powerful herb which is used to treat digestive problems. It is also capable of stimulating the digestive system, gallbladder and the liver. When taken internally, it is used to treat the following conditions:

- Anorexia

- Gastric infections

- Indigestion

- Liver complaints

Chapter 4: Know the Ten (10) Most Common Herb and Medicinal Garden Mistakes and How to Avoid Them

Common Mistake No. 1: Not applying any fertilizers.

Once you have herbs and medicinal plants planted and growing, it is very essential to keep them growing healthy with the use of a light, all purpose fertilizer. Apply a compost tea once every week to give your herbal and medicinal plants a boost. Herbs and medicinal plants are going to be harvested a lot of times during the growing season. This only means that your plants will be need an extra boost in order to keep their growth cycle for an extended time. When applying fertilizer, make sure to keep the soil hydrated and not the leaves themselves along with the compost tea. This practice will be healthier for the plant and contaminations in the leaves will also be avoided.

Common Mistake No. 2: Not protecting the plants enough.

While the herbal and medicinal plants are known to be hardy and resistant to diseases and bug problems, they can still arise. A lot of times, herbal and medicinal plant gardeners are scared to employ any strategy to safeguard their plants. This should not be the case. There are a lot of homemade and organic controls that are safe to use for edible herbal and medicinal plants. Organic gardening begins before the plant is even in place. Good soil and beneficial insects work altogether towards a chemical free herbal and medicinal garden.

Common Mistake No. 3: Not watering the plants properly

The needs of herbal and medicinal plants are very minimal. While they are very easy to maintain and care for, these plants will be providing you with fresh harvest all season. Herbal and medicinal plants however require proper watering schedule in order to remain free from stress.

Herbal and medicinal plants should be watered in the early morning, if possible. In this way, the water will soak deeper into the soil without having to deal with any evaporation issue. Always keep the soil around the plant hydrated and never water over the leaves as this will only promote diseases and mildews. Good mulch is important for your herbs as well. This will keep the soil hydrated and may extend the time between watering. Avoid mulching right next to the plant's stem though as this may invite insects and other types of invaders to make their home.

Common Mistake No. 4: Not paying attention to the tiny details.

It is a must to watch herbal and medicinal gardens closely. You need to know what the plant should look like while it is healthy as this will allow you to immediately notice when a problem first happens. Keep an eye on any damaged stems, leaves and disturbed soil around the plant. If you notice that the stems and leaves are beginning to fade, turn brown or curl up, you will have became aware of the problem early enough to possibly save the plant.

Common Mistake No. 4: Spraying chemical compounds into the plants

Herbs and medicinal plants are usually rinsed and used fresh. They should never be exposed to any kind of treatment that may possibly be toxic or dangerous to those who would eat them.

Even if a product claims that it is safe to use around pets and people, you should look for the words safe for edibles. You cannot rinse a bunch of basil leaves with water and soup prior to using. There are a lot of ways to keep ahead of the problems that may require the application of chemicals. Weed on a regular basis, watch the plants closely for any insect infestation and use natural fertilizers such as compost tea.

Common Mistake No. 5: Allowing the flowers to turn into seeds.

Herbal and medicinal plants grow beautiful flowers. While a lot of these plants have edible flowers, it is not a great idea to allow the herb to flower early during the growing season. Once your plant flowers, this signals that its life cycle is about to come into an end. Your plant is growing a flower, then a seed, then it dies back for that particular season.

It is a better idea to keep any blossoms from forming in the first place. When you see a flower about to grow, just pinch the entire thing off. You will notice that the plant may become persistent. In such case, cut the entire stem or below the flower.

Common Mistake No. 6: overcrowding or planting incorrectly

It is common to purchase more plants that you can possibly grow in a given area. When purchasing your herbal and medicinal plants, read the plant tags that usually come with each pot. Keep an eye to the width and height of the fully grown plant. You can always grow a quick growing annual between the plants, if you do not prefer the look of mulch. It is always a good idea to underplant rather than plant the herbs too close to each other from the beginning. Over planting is a big waste for money as it will not allow your plants to grow a healthy root system. A sturdy root system will help them survive the winter and expand the next growing season.

Common Mistake No. 7: Not cutting back enough

Pruning is what makes a plant to grow fast and neat. Pruning an herb implies that you are actually harvesting the good tasting stems and leaves. If you omit pruning, the plant will only tend to grow taller on a few stems. The leaves will grow old, dry and fall off. This will result to longer stems without leaves, Pruning will also allow the plant to begin and finish its life cycle. By regular pruning, you are actually keeping the plant in its growing phase for as long as possible. It will keep the flowers from budding, promotes leaves and stems and keeps the plant producing for an extended period of time. Your plants will appear healthier and better, if pruned back on a regular basis.

Common Mistake No. 9: Growing the plants in the wrong environment.

Are you growing rosemary, a chalky and dry loving plant in a humid and moist area? Your plant will surely die off in about 2 weeks from wet feet. If you would like to grow plants in a shady area, go for plants that can tolerate less sun. The sun=loving plants will grow weak and pale from not enough bright sunlight daily. If you have neither too shady nor too sunny area, try planting in pots that can be rolled or moved to the optimal lighting conditions. It is not a matter of sufficient shading or sun but is just a matter of finding a way to be adaptable to what you already have.

Common Mistake No. 10: Choosing unhealthy medicinal and herbal plants

The very first chance you have to find the perfect plant is when you actually buy it. Search for healthy plants, bright in color, plenty of foliage and certainly not one egg or bug on it. Finding a single aphid means that there are a lot more that you cannot see, all awaiting for the perfect time to invade your other plants. Never have the sympathy for a weak looking plant, unless you have a lot of space to keep it isolated from your main garden area while you try to repair the damage. The effort and time to be spent in repairing an infested herb garden means wasted time. Take the extra step to look for the healthiest plants that you can purchase.

Conclusion

Thank you again for purchasing this book!

I hope this book was able to help you to know how to successfully grow medicinal plants and herbs at home.

The next step is to follow the step-by-step guide and see your plants grow healthier each day.

Finally, if you enjoyed this book, please take the time to share your thoughts and post a review on Amazon. We do our best to reach out to readers and provide the best value we can. Your positive review will help us achieve that. It'd be greatly appreciated!

Thank you and good luck!

Check Out My Other Books

Below you'll find some of my other popular books that are popular on Amazon and Kindle as well. Simply click on the links below to check them out. Alternatively, you can visit my author page on Amazon to see other work done by me.

Coconut Oil for Easy Weight Loss

http://amzn.to/1i5f45p

Essential Oils & Aromatherapy

http://amzn.to/1ouuZTx

Superfoods that Kickstart Your Weight Loss

http://amzn.to/1eyHdku

The Best Secrets Of Natural Remedies

http://amzn.to/1gmHd7y

The Hypothyroidism Handbook

http://amzn.to/1emWfyR

The Hyperthyroidism Handbook

http://amzn.to/1kqLQCp

Essential Oils & Weight Loss For Beginners

http://amzn.to/Q83bFp

Essential Oils Box Set #33: Essential Oils & Aromatherapy for Beginners & The Beginners Guide to Medicinal Plants

Top Essential Oil Recipes

http://amzn.to/1lSrhSC

Soap Making For Beginners

http://amzn.to/1fkmYwr

Body Butters For Beginners

http://amzn.to/1fWjwJe

Homemade Body Scrubs & Masks For Beginners

http://amzn.to/1jjLRIO

Carrier Oils For Beginners

http://amzn.to/1sbqUQP

Natural Homemade Cleaning Recipes For Beginners

http://amzn.to/1izDB2m

The Beginners Guide To Medicinal Plants

http://amzn.to/1vSujr6

The Beginners Guide To Making Your Own Essential Oils

http://amzn.to/1piUNSB

The Beginners Alkaline Miracle Diet

http://amzn.to/1sDVaVE

Essential Oils Box Set #33: Essential Oils & Aromatherapy for Beginners & The Beginners Guide to Medicinal Plants

Thyroid Diet

http://amzn.to/1piW2RY

Essential Oils Box Set #1 (Weight Loss + Essential Oil Recipes

http://amzn.to/1qlYWWP

Essential Oils Box Set #2 (Weight Loss + Essential Oil & Aromatherapy

http://amzn.to/1qlYWWP

Essential Oils Box Set #3 Coconut Oil + Apple Cider Vinegar

http://amzn.to/1oIFZJw

Essential Oils Box Set #4 Body Butters & Top Essential Oil Recipes

http://amzn.to/1jSxURJ

Essential Oils Box Set #5 Soap Making & Homemade Body Scrubs

http://amzn.to/RAvJYo

Essential Oils Box Set #6 Body Butters & Body Scrubs

http://amzn.to/RAvSel

Essential Oils Box Set #7 Top Essential Oils & Best Kept Secrets Of Natural Remedies

http://amzn.to/1gvsRCq

Essential Oils Box Set #8 Homemade Cleaning Recipes & Essential Oil Recipes

http://amzn.to/1gxFAVb

Essential Oils Box Set #33: Essential Oils & Aromatherapy for Beginners & The Beginners Guide to Medicinal Plants

Essential Oils Box Set #9 Essential Oil and Weight Loss & Carrier Oils

http://amzn.to/1jmcEPP

Essential Oils Box Set #10 Hyperthyroidism Manual & Hypothyroidism Manual

http://amzn.to/1nHgJU4

Essential Oils Box Set #11 Carrier Oils for Beginners & Coconut Oil for Easy Weight Loss

http://amzn.to/1nHfy6X

Essential Oils Box Set #12 Essential Oils Weight Loss & Essential Oils Aromatherapy & Natural Homemade Cleaning Supplies & Top Essential Oil Recipes & Carrier Oils
http://amzn.to/1nHfy6X

Essential Oils Box Set #13 Superfoods & Essential Weight Loss & Essential Aromatherapy & Body Butters & Soap Making
http://amzn.to/1nUds6v

Essential Oils Box Set #14 Weight Loss & Apple Cider Vinegar & Body Butters & Homemade Body Scrubs & Coconut Oil for Beginners
http://amzn.to/1i1qYOd

If the links do not work, for whatever reason, you can simply search for these titles on the Amazon website to find them.

www.ingramcontent.com/pod-product-compliance
Lightning Source LLC
Chambersburg PA
CBHW070500290526
45790CB00003B/1029